The Little
Book of
Pilates

For Nikki

The Little
Book of
Pilates

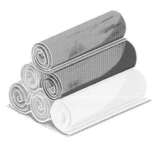

Una L. Tudor

An Hachette UK Company

www.hachette.co.uk

First published in Great Britain in 2022
by Gaia, an imprint of
Octopus Publishing Group Ltd
Carmelite House
50 Victoria Embankment
London EC4Y 0DZ

www.octopusbooks.co.uk

Distributed in the US by Hachette
Book Group
1290 Avenue of the Americas
4th and 5th Floors
New York, NY 10104

Distributed in Canada by
Canadian Manda Group
664 Annette St.
Toronto, Ontario,
Canada M6S 2C8

ISBN 978-1-85675-443-9

A CIP catalogue record for this book is
available from the British Library.

Printed and bound in China

10 9 8 7 6 5 4 3 2 1

Publisher: Lucy Pessell
Editor: Sarah Kennedy
Designer: Hannah Coughlin
Illustrator: Abi Read
Copy Editor: Jane Birch
Proofreader: Clare Churly
Production Controller: Emily Noto

Contents

Introduction

In the late Victorian era, in the German city of Gladbach, there was a sickly little boy. His name was Joseph Pilates, and he suffered from asthma, rickets and rheumatic fever. If he had had different parents, he might have lived very differently: he might have been wrapped up in cotton wool or kept always indoors or told to save his strength. But Joseph's father, a Greek metalworker, was an enthusiastic amateur gymnast. And he believed – must have believed – that his son could do anything. He must have believed that his son's thin, wheezing little body was capable of greatness. The father took his son to gymnastics with him; he had Joseph taught not only bodybuilding, but boxing and jiu-jitsu too. Plus, when we say gymnastics, we're not just talking about jumping and balancing (although that matters too). At this time, gymnastics also included what we would now call weightlifting and strength training: there's a picture of the father holding his heavy barbells, posing. And he wasn't the only one. Joseph posed too. By the time he was 14, the definition of his muscles was textbook, and Joseph was the model for anatomical charts.

It's not surprising, then, that Joseph grew up to be a personal trainer. In fact, he moved to England, where he trained

Scotland Yard in self-defence. In his spare time, he was a professional boxer...and a circus strongman! But when the First World War broke out, Joseph, like every other German in England, was detained in an internment camp, in Joseph's case on the Isle of Man. Left without any policemen to train, audiences to show off for or equipment to work with, Joseph started thinking. It must have seemed to Joseph that, without the sports that had saved him, he was in danger of returning to his childhood self: sickly and afraid. And everyone around him was in the same boat.

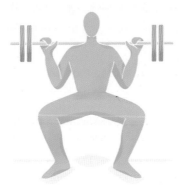

Inspired by Cats

And so Joseph devised a system. He was inspired by yoga, and his own sporting history – and the movement of cats he saw around the place. (He liked cats.) He trained himself in this system, which required nothing but dedication and time, and he began to train others too. This system had such good results that they even began to send Joseph the wounded veterans for rehabilitation. Out of the trauma of war, Joseph managed to create something wonderful: a space for healing, and a place to find strength, flexibility and compassion. A system, in short, that allowed Joseph to have control over not only his own body, but his routine and his world.

We, of course, call it Pilates, after the man who founded it.

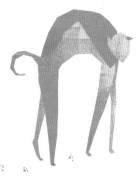

There are six principles of Pilates:

• Breath

• Concentration

• Control

• Precision

• Centre

• Flow

This Little Book has six chapters, one dedicated to each of these principles – both in Pilates and in life. The founding idea of Pilates is to unite mind and body as one, not only in the moment we take these exercises, but in every other moment too. We study Pilates not just as a form of exercise, but as a way of life. By taking these six principles as the principles of our being, we become stronger, healthier, happier people.

The Importance of Order

Joseph Pilates instructed that there was a very clear order in which his exercises should be performed. He believed very strongly that the sequence of exercises was almost as important as the exercises themselves. There are 34 exercises in total, some easy, some difficult, and traditionally they must be performed in the correct order. Joseph's *Return to Life Through Contrology* runs to many pages, with detailed descriptions of each exercise – but it's always best to find a qualified teacher or someone who can help you. On the opposite page you'll find the complete list of exercises in order. While we can only show a few sketches, online or in a studio you'll find many helpful videos to bring that precision and focus that Pilates demands.

This book touches upon some of the easier exercises in Pilates to give you a flavour of what it can do – and what it can do for you. I have chosen the simpler exercises to make sure you're able to succeed at home, and to succeed only with the equipment you will definitely have available to you (a floor!).

Joseph's 34 Exercises

1. *Hundred*
2. *Roll Up*
3. *Roll Over*
4. *One Leg Circle*
5. *Rolling Like a Ball*
6. *Single Leg Stretch*
7. *Double Leg Stretch*
8. *Spine Stretch*
9. *Rocker with Open Legs*
10. *Corkscrew*
11. *Saw*
12. *Swan-dive*
13. *One Leg Kick*
14. *Double Leg Kick*
15. *Neck Pull*
16. *Scissors*
17. *Bicycle*

18. *Shoulder Bridge*
19. *Spine Twist*
20. *Jack Knife*
21. *Side Kick*
22. *Teaser*
23. *Hip Twist*
24. *Swimming*
25. *Leg Pull – Front*
26. *Leg Pull*
27. *Side Kick Kneeling*
28. *Side Bend*
29. *Boomerang*
30. *Seal*
31. *Crab*
32. *Rocking*
33. *Control Balance*
34. *Push Up*

When practising the exercises, you may find it helpful to record yourself reading them on your phone or a voice recorder, so you can play the instructions back to yourself during the exercises.

It's worth noting that many teachers have developed their own order in the many decades since Joseph's death – and it's also worth noting that how you feel is important too. Perhaps you don't have time in the day to follow every instruction in Joseph's manual – and that's okay. This has to work for you, and your life.

And yet – could you make the time? When you look into your core self, do you want to make the time to do this? Could you, if you really focused, make space for a little time for the self?

If so, you'll find something magic happens: when performed together, the exercises somehow flow into each other: you always end up in the right place for the next one to start.

This, of course, is the genius of Pilates: with a system that always, always reconnects us to the core, we will always be poised for the next thing. When we are aware of our core, and conscious of our breath, we will always be ready for whatever happens next.

But let's take it right back to the beginning. Let's move through the exercises in this book together, and begin… with a single breath.

Chapter 1: Breath

> Above all,
> learn to breathe
>
> – Joseph Pilates

Let's start with a breath: a deep, cleansing sigh of a breath.

Breathe in. Breathe out.

Maybe this isn't where you expected this book to begin.
Maybe you thought we'd get straight into the poses. And we
will – we'll get to that. But first let's start with a breath. Let's
start with the breath, and how it feels.

Notice the Breath

Stand or sit comfortably, with your shoulders back. Kiss your shoulder blades together, if you can, and find stillness — whatever that looks like to you.

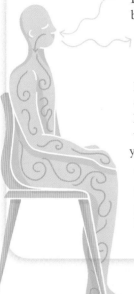

Breathe. Breathe in, and breathe out.

Notice your breath, without judgement or fear. There is no wrong answer here; this is simply an observation exercise. We are looking for your baseline: we are trying to find your "normal".

What do we send out into the world? And what do we pull in? How do we give, and how do we take? This might

seem like a lot to put on a single, simple breath —
but that's okay. This is just a starting point. A safe
place to stand and observe yourself.

Ask yourself:

- How does the breath feel in my mouth and my
  nose? How about in my chest?

- How does the breath feel in my lungs? Is it
  reaching every part of my lungs, or just the top?

- How does the breath feel in my throat? Is it cold
  or hot? Does it hurt at all?

- How does my body feel when I breathe in? How
  does my body feel when I breathe out?

- How does it sound? How does it taste? How
  does it smell? If something hurts, notice it. If
  something feels good, notice it.

Look. Listen. Observe. Be kind with yourself; be
patient. There are no wrong answers here. You
cannot get this wrong. I promise!

You might be wondering why we didn't try to modulate the breath here at all: why, if something hurt, I didn't ask you to change it, or fix it; why there are no instructions for fixing a ragged breath, or deepening a shallow breath. Maybe you think: what's the point in looking at things if we aren't going to work on fixing them?

And yet, I promise you, we will get to fixing things – but we can't fix anything if we don't know what's wrong. We know that something is definitely wrong...and we know that because you've picked up this book.

You want to make a change. You want something to be different in yourself – and maybe you don't even know what that is yet.

Unlike a lot of exercise regimes (and for that matter, therapeutic programmes), Pilates doesn't separate out the mind from the body. That's why people come to Pilates for all sorts of reasons, mental and physical, in need of all kinds of healing – and sometimes the thing they think they're coming to fix isn't the thing they needed to fix at all.

You see, all efforts for self-improvement begin with an increased consciousness. Think of that sense, perhaps, that you could be doing something better, or that you could be feeling better: that sense that something isn't working the way you want it to. The trouble is, too often that increased consciousness isn't working for us: it's working against us. We notice the flaws in our bodies and the gaps in our knowledge: all the ways we don't live up to an invented ideal. Are the flaws we see even real? Are they the flaws anyone else would notice about us? Are we holding ourselves to impossible standards?

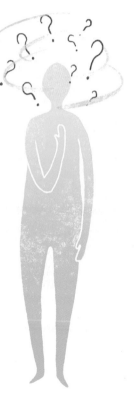

We're all already bringing with us, into this Little Book, a hyper-aware state. And it might be getting in the way. This breathing exercise we've just done is really an exercise in consciousness: rechannelling the hyper-awareness that drove us here into an increased self-knowledge.

Consciousness is at the heart of wellbeing – and at the heart of Pilates.

Applying Consciousness

As we saw in the Introduction, there are six pillars of Pilates, set down by the disciples of Joseph Pilates to simplify his original system, in order to make it more accessible. Those pillars form the six chapters of this book: breath, concentration, control, precision, centre and flow. If you think about it, those six words could be further simplified down to "consciousness".

Breath: *be conscious of the start of it all.*

Concentration: *be conscious of where your attention wanders.*

Control: *be conscious of the power we have, and how we use it.*

Precision: *be conscious of your words and actions and movements.*

Centre: *be conscious of where we come from, and how we move.*

Flow: *be conscious of the sequence of our movements, and ourselves.*

Breathe; concentrate; take control.

Be precise; move strongly and decisively from your centre; move smoothly with flow.

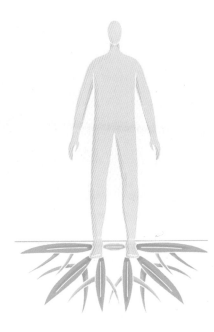

Pilates, done right, will give you not only what you want but what you really need. It does this by giving you the space to figure out what it is that's bothering you, and the tools to take charge of putting it right.

We apply this increased consciousness to our bodies and minds; we practise daily through Pilates; and we find ourselves more attuned to the world.

We find ourselves more able to move through life with strength and dignity. We find the places in our mind and body that are stiff or sore; and find the edges of our competence and comfort. We find the shape of who we are in order to find what we'd like to change.

So let's see what we can change, before we begin anything to do with Pilates proper at all. Let's see what small changes can have a big difference in the way we feel.

And we start, of course, with breath.

Sama Vritti Breath (Taking Control)

This exercise is drawn from an ancient Sanskrit practice called *pranayama*: if you've ever practised yoga, you'll be familiar with this word. It means "life force" (*prana*) plus "extended" (*yama*). It refers to the act of breathing correctly. We are going to modulate our breath, now, in accordance with one of the simplest *pranayama*: *sama vritti*, meaning "same action". Each in-breath, and each out-breath, will become the same. So:

Sit or lie down comfortably.

Place your hands on your rib cage, gently tucked around your waist – you should be able to feel the

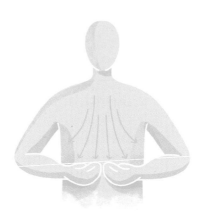

bottom of your ribs under your palms. Bring that attention to your breath here, as before: just notice.

Start a count in your head: in-two-three-four-five, out-two-three-four-five. Count evenly, neither too fast nor too slow.

Bring your breath in line with the count: in for five, and out for five. Don't gulp the air down or huff it out. Try to keep the breaths steady and even: you want each beat, ideally, to be the same pace and tempo and force as the others.

You can check in with your shoulders here to get a good idea of whether you're keeping the beat steady: do they rise and fall evenly? What about your hands, balanced on your ribs? Are they rising and falling?

As you even out your breath, try to – sort of – push it down under your hands. Breathe into your cupped palms. Fill them with air as your lungs expand; and hollow them out as your lungs contract. A good thing to focus on here is the idea of "working smarter not harder": you don't need more air, you just need the air you already have to fill the lungs evenly and smoothly.

You see: already we're getting into flow, into control, into concentration and precision and breathing from the centre. Joseph Pilates knew that everything started with breath, and it's only once we've mastered that that we can start to explore further…

Chapter 2: Concentration

Concentrate on the
correct movement

– Joseph Pilates

Pilates is a system of correct movements.

It is a system of precise, small muscular movements that – taken together – allow you to take full control of your body. It aims to strengthen the body evenly, so that one part doesn't take undue precedence over the other. Each muscle works at peak performance alongside all the others, in absolute harmony. The improvements in muscle tone balance each other out, and it is this balance that allows us to improve posture and joint mobility. When we can rely on each muscle to work for the benefit of the others, nothing is overtaxed – and nothing is underused and slack. It is, essentially, a collaborative system where every collaborator is you. Pilates is about making sense of your body as a united whole – and your mind too.

It makes sense, right? When things go wrong in the body, it's because things have become unbalanced. There's too much of something or too little of something; one bit is doing too much or too little. Things are tilted too far one way.

This is science, rather than spirituality: think of cancer cells multiplying much too much and much too fast, for instance. Or, more prosaically, a sore neck when we've been carrying a bag on one shoulder for too long. Or a sore back when we've been sitting hunched over a laptop, physically unbalancing ourselves. Or even a sore mind when we've been dwelling on one thing for too long. Too much is concentrated on too little, and it throws us off.

If we don't notice this imbalance, it just goes on getting worse. We have to notice. We have to pay attention to the places where our bodies and minds are screaming out for attention, and we have to treat them with care.

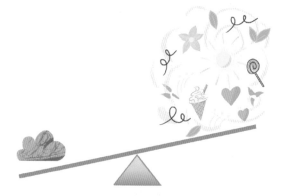

Finding a Neutral Spine

Let's take a moment here to find our "neutral spine". This is crucial in Pilates, because the neutral spine is different for everyone – and it's very hard to achieve in the modern world. Joseph Pilates felt that the modern world was ruining our bodies by making us contort over desks – and he was born long before the rise of the laptop!

We find our neutral spine so that we can set our own default, and find where we've been literally, physically unbalanced.

A neutral spine is just one that you're not contorting in any way.

The neutral spine is a spine that takes into account all the natural curves of the back. There are three of these curves: neck, middle and lower, or cervical, thoracic and lumbar if you want to be fancy. A neutral spine also isn't overextended or twisted in any way.

You'll probably find, when lying flat, that there are two spaces where your back doesn't touch the floor: probably at your neck and under your lower back.

So how do we figure out what our neutral spine should look like? What's our neutral, natural state?

We find it, of course, through mindful awareness.

We lie flat on the floor, and breathe deep. Five in, five out.

Tuck your shoulder blades beneath you, and tuck in your core muscles.

With your hands, form a triangle (thumb to thumb, index finger to index finger) and rest that triangle pointing down on the stomach, with the index fingers above the pubic bone.

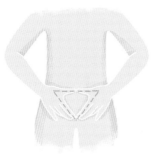

Now, inhale, and on the exhale, tilt the pelvis so that the triangle is pointing up to the sky. Inhale, and tilt the other way, so that the triangle points down. (This is, of course, only a guide; it won't literally point up or down!)

Repeat this rocking motion, and notice: notice how your spine feels.

Settle against the floor, comfortably. Notice what touches the floor and what doesn't. This is your neutral spine. This will be your default starting place for the exercises in this book.

Being Fully Present

This is concentration, yes, but it's also mindfulness.

The American Psychological Association defines mindfulness as a "moment-to-moment awareness of one's experience without judgement", which is a pretty good way of looking at it. It's about being fully present, in both your body and the space it inhabits, and it's a natural state of being. I mean this. We all know how it feels to be engaged and interested in something – so mindfulness is about bringing that engagement into our everyday lives. It's about being interested in the smallest possible sensations of living, right here, right now. It's about accepting and acknowledging all that comes with that interest.

It has also become something of a buzz word in the last decade. You may even be switching off just thinking about it. You may have been directed to mindfulness by a doctor, a therapist or even your employer. It has been touted as a kind of "cure-all" – often without proper support.

This is very wrong. Mindfulness isn't a craze, but a way of living that we can combine with other things (like Pilates) to help us understand what we're giving of ourselves, and how.

This is not some frivolous millennial idea. Rather, it's based on ancient Zen Buddhist principles about living in the moment – and about paying attention to that moment. It's about not being distracted by the future, or weighed down by the past, but understanding where we belong in the now. It is about finding your own edges, and how those edges blur into the universe: an intense concentration on the self that allows us to bring our attention to everything else as well.

Let's continue this focus chapter with a mindfulness exercise.

Full Body Scan

For this one, let's lie down. Settle yourself comfortably into place.

Start by taking a mental temperature check. How do you feel about doing this exercise? Do you feel silly or fidgety or self-indulgent? Is your mind full of thoughts? (Don't worry if it is. We're thought-producing machines, and this isn't Zen Buddhism. Over the course of the next few chapters, we're going to do the kind of work that drives all other thoughts out anyway!)

Then, notice your breathing. Bring it, once again, into that five-five shape (see page 25). In for five, and out for five. Feel how it fills the body; feel how it empties.

Feel the breath moving through the body: the mouth, the throat, the chest, the diaphragm. We've already done this, so this shouldn't feel too weird or new to you. The attention we bring to the breath is the exact same attention we're going to need in this chapter: attention, focus and concentration are all really other words for consciousness.

So let's try it: bring that close attention to the places your body touches the bed or sofa or floor. How does it feel? How do you feel?

This is a big question, so let's draw it into the very littlest of loci: your little toes. How do they feel? Maybe you've never contemplated your little toes before – unless they hurt! – but now you can. Bring the attention into your other toes, too: your toes, arches, heels, ankles.

Move very slowly up the legs, through calves and knees and thighs and hips.

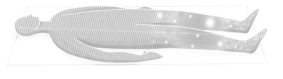

I like to picture it like a green light, moving up through and illuminating each section of bone and muscle and skin and tendon: concentrating and examining with the breath. What colour light would you like to work with? I picture this grass-green colour for examining, and a warm pink for healing, and perhaps a soft yellow for clarity. This is your exercise, so try visualizing whatever colour makes you happiest.

Let the breath be the guide; whenever we feel our attention creeping away, bring the breath back to that steady five-five time. As we breathe, we concentrate; and then we can move that concentration (and maybe our visualized light, if we chose to try that) up through our feet into our legs, and from our legs into our torso: back, belly, chest, noticing any sensations or even emotions. Concentrate. Visualize. Change nothing; just note, and feel. Your feelings and sensations are valid and real. Breathe in, breathe out.

Pull your attention through the chest and lungs, and send it down each arm, your biceps and triceps, elbows, forearms, hands and fingers and fingertips, and all the way back up again across the shoulders.

You might want to focus here on the shoulder blades and perhaps check back in with the spine, both of which can get pretty achy at times. How's it feeling?

Breathe in, breathe out. From the shoulders, move into the neck, and the hollow of the throat inside and out. Trace it up to your chin, mouth, nose, cheeks. Notice any pressure in your jaw or temples. Notice any pain or strain. Notice how your eyes

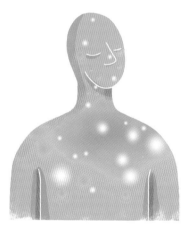

feel; your ears; even your scalp. Bring your attention to something as small as the hair follicles on your head: maybe you wear your hair in a ponytail or bun, and actually, it's starting to hurt. These small pains have worth; they deserve to be noticed. Just like the rest of you.

When you're ready, open your eyes. Give yourself a moment or two to notice the world around you: does it seem the same as before? Do you feel the same as before?

So concentration, focus and mindfulness are all drawing from the same well. But what are the benefits? Why do this at all?

Supported by Science

The benefits of mindful thinking are myriad, and backed up by science. Many, many studies have shown that mindfulness makes people less sad, less stressed and less afraid. Which are, of course, the things we're all hoping for when we pick up a book like this. We've all come to Pilates (or any other form of self-help) looking for a change in the way we feel – and this mindful thinking is scientifically proven to do so. In 2010, a behavioural scientist named Stefan G. Hoffman[1] wrote a paper that summed up almost 40 other studies into the effects of mindfulness on the body. He looked at people with depression, with anxiety, with cancer and a whole range of other health conditions – and how mindfulness had helped or not helped their sense of wellbeing. He found that there was "robust" evidence to suggest that it was "effective" on all of these kinds of problems.

A 2006 study, published in the journal *American Psychologist*[2], found that training yourself to have this kind of focus increased "calmness, clarity and concentration". It increases your metacognitive abilities and your memory – and those two things together allow you to have greater emotional control. Greater emotional control means that you're less likely to find yourself in a spiral of shame or panic or unhappiness; and you're better able to manage your relationships with others and with yourself.

Actually, when you think about it, the benefits of everything from psychotherapy to palm reading come down to taking the time to mindfully look at yourself and your life.

While Joseph Pilates never used the word itself, "mindfulness" – consciousness – is at the heart of his exercise regime. That is where the balance comes from: knowing yourself right down to the last muscle. You have to allow yourself to feel in each muscle how it moves, how it works and how it is supposed to work.

So with that in mind, let's come to the first actual Pilates exercise: Imprinting (see page 46). For the Pilates exercises in this book, you might want to look up videos or ask a friend/ instructor to show you the correct form if you're unsure.

While many kinds of Pilates use machines, like Reformer Pilates, every exercise in this book can be done at home on a yoga mat. I strongly advise that machine Pilates must be taught by an instructor, so that you can make sure you are using the equipment properly and safely, even if you would like to practise the exercises in this book alone at home – but you should always check with your doctor if you have any concerns at all.

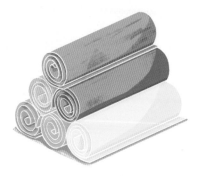

EXERCISE

Imprinting

Imprinting is the first thing we learn in Pilates, and it's very simple.

We bring ourselves into that neutral spine position (see page 31), knees up, feet flat on the floor, arms by our sides, and we relax. Yes. I know it's surprising.

Relax every muscle in the body; all those muscles we've just observed in the body scan on page 36. Use only the energy you need to keep your knees up and feet flat. Tuck your core in, but without too much effort: think of it just like tidying up. A

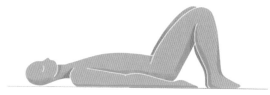

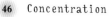

folding and rearranging, rather than a tight squeeze.

Visualize your ribs touching the floor, and visualize your hips settling into the floor too. Visualize your nice neutral spine melting into the floor. Sometimes it helps to imagine that the floor is made of something spongy, like a memory-foam mattress, and that you are actually nestling into it like a little bird settling down for the night.

Visualize your spine settling down into the softness, and see if you can imagine the line it leaves there. This is the imprint we are talking about. Breathe into the imprint. Breathe out. Inhale for five, and exhale for five.

Settle yourself. From this neutral spine and imprinted position, we can tackle every single one of the Pilates positions we'll encounter in this Little Book...and so, so many more. This book only gives a flavour of what we can do together.

Chapter 3: Control

> Be in control of your body and not at its mercy
>
> – Joseph Pilates

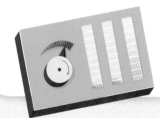

When we practise Pilates, we're bringing the mind in line with the body. The chaos of the universe is also the chaos of the mind, and by simplifying everything right down, we strip that chaos back. We are, at last, making the mental thoughts match up with the physical self. We have harmony between mind and body, between breath and movement. We are present in our bodies in a way that allows us to be present in the moment, located firmly in space and time.

You Own Your Body

You see, anxiety is often not about what's in front of us but what we imagine might be coming soon. It's not about what's really there, but what isn't: what we might have to do, what might be done to us, what might happen in the

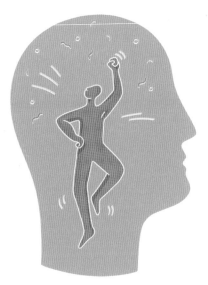

wide and scary world. And it's not that those fears aren't real. It's just that there is often nothing we can do about them. Actually, if we could do something about them, we'd feel less afraid. It's the powerlessness that hurts so much – and so by owning the only power we ever really have, we combat that panic before it begins.

There are so few things in this universe that we can control, and maybe – just maybe – our bodies could be one of them. Pilates can be adapted by bodies of all kinds, and this message – that your body is your own and you are in charge of it – is one for every single human being on this earth.

Our bodies are the only things we can ever truly own. They are the only things over which we can expect always to have total dominion; the only possession that literally cannot be taken from us and to which nobody else, ever, for any reason has a claim. Your body is your own. My body is my own. To claim that for ourselves is a radical and vital act.

"Contrology"

Think of the beginnings of Pilates as mentioned earlier in this book; think of all the soldiers who had been told their bodies belonged to the state, to use and abuse as they pleased; and all the citizens kept in internment camps, physically moved and removed from their homes and settled lives. Think of Joseph, taken from a trusted job teaching the forces of the state, and then compelled by those same forces to be under their control. This is a system designed to restore a sense of power to the self. This is a system designed to restore you to you.

It was all about control: giving back a little control to those people who had had their lives stolen from them, and restoring some control to those returning soldiers who had had their bodies changed and damaged by the ravages of war.

Joseph even called the system "Contrology" (before it was later renamed Pilates), to keep this idea at the heart of everything he did.

Taking Control

Psychologists like Bessel van der Kelk, author of the much-beloved resource *The Body Keeps the Score*[3], believe that Pilates has a vital role to play in patients suffering from even the most extreme post-traumatic stress disorder (PTSD). Trauma like this is essentially dissociative. "This can't be happening," we think, and our minds decide, sometimes, that perhaps it isn't.

You've heard, maybe, of people saying that they felt that they left their body in an event like a car crash – and it's that that we're discussing here. There is a gap between the normal self, and the self that this happened to. There is a gap between the

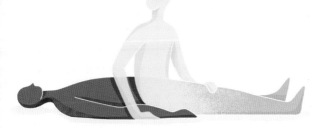

physical person we used to be, and the physical person we are now; a gap between the physical person who is suffering and the physical person who had suffered; a gap between the intellectual knowledge that we have suffered, the physical marks of that suffering, and the emotional self in denial.

When we come to Pilates, we bring all that with us. And perhaps this doesn't resonate with you on a major level: perhaps it feels like too strong a term for what you've been through. But trauma happens in many ways, big and small. Perhaps you had a difficult birth, or narrowly escaped being hurt, or saw someone you loved get sick and die. Perhaps someone you loved let you down in a way you can't stop thinking about. Perhaps you have blamed yourself for something that wasn't your fault. Now, Pilates isn't therapy – but it can be hugely therapeutic.

We bring all this baggage with us wherever we go. We might wonder how we'd start to set it down, but Pilates doesn't ask us to do that. It doesn't ask us to let go of what we're bringing. It's often not possible to escape our past, any more than Joseph Pilates could escape the internment camp he lived in or the soldiers could erase the horrors of combat.

But it does give us a space to work with that heaviness. The body as it is, and the mind as it is, must come together; and we must be in control of both. We control the body with the mind, but we also bring the mind in line with what we physically need. We have come to Pilates because we felt a physical need to stretch and twist and bend, and the intellectual mind just has to come along too. It's impossible to do Pilates properly without thinking about it: we have to exercise that concentration in order to have control.

And once we have control over the body, we start to feel as if we have a little more control over our own lives too.

The following exercise will help you hone in on the "control" element of Pilates.

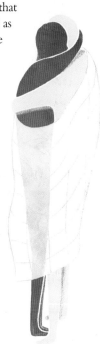

Pelvic Curl

Lie flat on your back. Breathe in for five; breathe out for five; breathe in again.

On the inhale, bend your knees so that your feet are flat on the floor, about a hip-width apart.

Arms lie flat on the mat either side of your torso, stretched out long.

Tuck your shoulder blades underneath you, and engage your core.

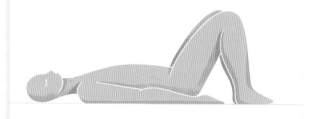

Exhale. Inhale. Exhale, and on that exhale gently squeeze your abdominal muscles together, drawing your pelvis underneath you. This is kind of a neat feeling: a tight, organized neatness in the abs.

Engaging your glutes, begin to roll up through the spine, peeling your back from the mat one vertebra at a time. Really focus on the order here. Each vertebra should leave the mat in order, until your body is a straight line from bent knee to resting shoulders.

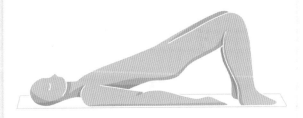

Inhale for five, keeping the body as steady and still as you can, and on the exhale, release.

Release with care, one vertebra at a time.

The crucial thing here is control: no sudden movements, no jerky movements, just a smooth, careful flow. You are the master of your vertebrae. Your spine is not the boss of your mind.

Repeat ten times, taking note of any tightness or difficulty you experience.

You might have noticed, following the exercise on the previous page, that it's very difficult to think of anything else when you're focusing on your vertebrae in this way.

Which is, of course, part of the point – and part of the reason that Pilates is so helpful in coping with stress, anxiety, depression and other traumatic circumstances. It works on multiple levels.

First, and most simply, if you're committing your mind completely to exercising conscious control over these tiny bones, there's no space left for anything else. When we occupy our mind with the very real activity of the body, we leave little space for endless, maddening what-ifs. Our thoughts are tied to the physical self, and our control over that physical self.

Secondly, by focusing completely on just that one little vertebra in a universe of chaos, we're actually coming close to something like mindfulness – or even something like Zen Buddhism. Think of how a monk in meditation might focus on a candle flame or a mantra. Your spine is the mantra. Your body is your flame.

Chapter 4: Precision

> Every moment of our life can be the beginning of great things
>
> – Joseph Pilates

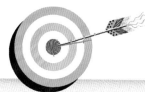

Every moment is a new moment. Every moment, we have a new chance to begin again. Every day we are given the chance to start trying to be the kind of people we want to be: people who are kinder, people who eat better or exercise more or achieve their dreams. Whatever it is you want, today – right here, right now – is a chance to strive for it.

This might feel terrifying.

Maybe this makes you feel inadequate, or like you aren't ready to become the person you want to be. If you could start now, why wouldn't you? Why haven't you? What's gone wrong?

The answer to all these questions, of course, is that you're human. You're human, and you're trying now, and that's all that really matters.

And when you fail (not if, but when, because we all fail) there's another minute, and another fresh start. There are infinite fresh starts. Joseph Pilates famously believed that a person's physical and mental peak should be in their seventies, and that old age didn't begin until you hit one hundred years old. There's enough time for you, reading this, to begin again right now. Right here, in this precise moment, we're going to begin again together. And – what's more – we're going to enjoy it.

Roll Like a Ball

The best thing about this exercise is just how much
fun it is: it introduces an element of childlike play
into serious exercise.

As a bonus, it gives the spine a real massage too.

It is very simple to perform, and you're probably
already familiar with the basic motion.

Sit up on your mat, and bring your knees into
your chest. Take a moment here to just hold
yourself; give yourself a big hug. Love yourself.
Nourish yourself.

Tuck in your core muscles, and bring your shoulder
blades together.

Then, open up the knees, still holding your legs, and lift your feet up off the mat. Bring your head between your knees, and balance here for a second.

Start to rock back and forth, as if you're soothing yourself gently – just a little at first, but then faster, and in rhythm. Rock back onto your shoulder blades, and back up to touch your feet to the mat.

Have fun with this exercise! Rock and roll! Feel what you feel!

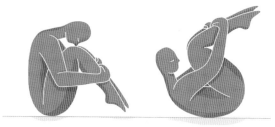

Changing Yourself
for the Better

Perhaps you're surprised to find this rolling-like-a-ball
exercise in the chapter on Precision. Certainly, it's not
ostensibly one of the more precise exercises in Pilates (and
we will be doing those too – don't you worry!). But we'll
start this chapter with rolling like a ball because it's fun.
Because it's a chance to move your body in a way that feels
fresh and a little silly and a little exciting. It starts the blood
moving and promotes deep breathing in a way that brings
energy and joy into the day. It brings us very physically into
the present moment – nobody can take themselves too
seriously when they are "rolling like a ball" – which allows
us to be here, with the precise body that we have, in the
precise place we are in, at the precise moment of deciding
to change.

Precision, in Pilates, usually refers to making sure every exercise is performed absolutely correctly. That's one reason I urge you to take a class, or at a minimum check out some videos online; I can't help you with your movements from here, and in Pilates it is the shapes we create with our bodies that matter so much. Each "well-designed" movement, as Joseph Pilates put it modestly, involves many tiny movements of muscles, and it is the balance of those movements together that make Pilates such an effective mental and physical workout.

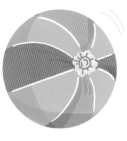

It also refers, of course, to that concentration and control we have discussed in the previous chapters – and none of these things can be achieved without precise and conscious control over the breath. A precise body is a controlled body; and a controlled body is a conscious body; and a conscious body working with a conscious mind allows you to be the master of your own destiny and fate. Precision implies, always, intent. When we intend to do something and then do it, we prove to ourselves (and others!) that we are capable of change. And we are capable of change.

We are capable of changing both ourselves, and our lives, for the better. And we can do that in this moment.

Every moment allows us to take a little step (a little rock, a little roll) toward the person we'd like to be, whatever that looks like to us.

Leg Circles

This is a great one for practising precision, because it's so easy to feel when you're going off balance.

Lie flat on the mat. This time, instead of arms by your sides, send them out horizontally, perpendicular to the body, like a T-shape.

Engage the core as always, tucking the pelvic muscles and tightening the abdominals, and send the left leg out long. Press the heel and the back of the shin into the mat; feel the ground supporting your back, glutes and thigh.

Exhale. Curl the right leg in toward the chest, and then straighten it up, up, up into the sky, as straight as you can manage, with your foot turned as if you were going to walk upside down. Imagine balancing something on the sole of your foot.

Inhale, and find stillness.

Then start to draw big, steady circles in the air with your foot – imagine a pen is held directly upright between your toes. Keep that circle smooth, precise and easy. If you start to wobble, just make the circle a little smaller.

Five circles clockwise, on the exhale; then inhale, find stillness, and, exhaling, draw five the other way.

Gently and with control, bring the right leg back down to the chest, and stretch out to join the left. Inhale. Find stillness, and draw the left leg up to the chest, exactly as before.

Five circles. Five circles. Inhale. Exhale.

Come to stillness lying on your back, and pause for a moment. Allow yourself this moment to reflect on what you intended to do, and how well you achieved it.

We're going to come straight now into another exercise.
Chest lifts are a core move for Pilates because they feature in
so many other exercises, and because they make such marked
improvements to both your muscle tone and your posture.
This particular exercise is also wonderful for those with neck
pain, back pain and even
headaches. When we
strengthen the muscles
around the spine, the
spine is more free, and less
contorted. (As ever, if you
have any concerns or feel
that anything is not right
with either neck or back,
please consult your
medical practitioner
before beginning!)

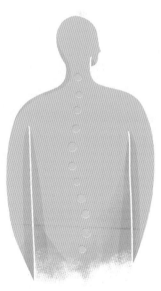

EXERCISE

Chest Lift

Lie on your back, with a nice neutral spine. Think of your imprint; and think too about your breath. In for five, out for five. Your knees should be bent, and your feet flat on the floor.

Your knees should line up with your hips, and your ankles should line up with your knees. We call this stacking because the bones are stacked on top of one another.

Bring your hands behind your head, to cradle your neck. Interlace the fingers. Look for your elbows at the edges of your peripheral vision.

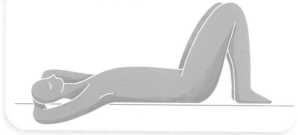

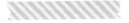

Elbows wide; shoulders down. Inhale. Exhale, and on the exhale pull the belly button down even further. Imagine that you are trying to print your belly button onto the mat through your spine – mad, but it works. Lengthen the spine.

Tilt your chin slightly down, as if you're cradling an egg between your chin and chest.

As you lengthen the spine, raise your upper body: your arms, your neck, your shoulders, your chin, your chest. Lead with the chest, and let everything else follow.

Lift, and come to a 45-degree angle from the mat: your shoulder blades should just leave the mat. Pause. Inhale, and exhale to slowly release.

Repeat five times.

Chapter 5:
Centre

True happiness, it is said, comes from within.

It can't be bought with money (although lack of money can certainly contribute to a lack of happiness!), and nor is it as simple as a question of deserving it. Plenty of people deserve happiness and never find it; plenty of people have no right to be half as happy as they are.

"Happiness," Charlotte Brontë so memorably wrote, "is not a potato." She meant that happiness could not be cultivated, but that it is simply a kind of blessing that shines down upon you from some exterior force. This is all very well if you have the kind of life that does shine down happiness on you at regular intervals – or if you're a miserable woman in a Gothic novel. For the rest of us, however, waiting for this kind of *deus ex machina* might make for a pretty grim time.

Waiting rooms are terrible places at the best of times – so why let our lives become so?

Learning to Be Happy

We have to make our happiness because the world is hard and nobody is going to do it for us; we have to become the kind of people we want to be, and build the kind of world we want to have. Happiness is work, and learning to be happy is work. Brains love patterns, and it's hard to break out of the pattern of misery once we find ourselves in it. And yet, you can do it. I know you can do it, because you're here, reading this book, and trying – and trying to be happy is the best start possible.

You're not only trying to be happy, you're trying to be healthy – in body and mind.

And you're trying, too, to find out what's wrong and how you can fix it. You're trying to listen to your body more, to hear better, to take notice of yourself. And I know this is true, because you've turned to Pilates and Pilates is all about that core, inner self.

The principle guiding this chapter is the word "centre", and I want you to think about that for a moment. Two questions to ask:

1. What is at the centre of my life?

2. What is at the centre of my self?

You might want to make some notes here if this sparks anything for you – just to scribble down some ideas or phrases that come into your head. The focus, in Pilates, on the centre allows us to open up a dialogue with the self: to know ourselves better. It is only through true self-knowledge that we can even begin to understand what makes us happy, and why; it is only through the control, focus and precision we have practised in previous chapters that we can then take and use that information to improve our lives and choices and bodies.

Sit with your answers to those questions for a moment. Do your answers make you happy? Is that what you hoped to find at the centre? Are those centres authentic? More than that, do they match? If, for instance, work is at the centre of your life; but there is a wanderlust at the centre of your soul, does that mismatch cause you suffering? Could you change anything there?

Remember everything we've said about balance and imbalance. Remember that the mind/body disconnect is in and of itself a traumatizing experience. Everything in this book has been in the hope of bringing the physical and mental into better alignment and that includes your goals and life and happiness.

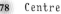

The First Requisite
of Happiness

Pilates is not just about the body, but about the ways improving the health of the body can improve the health of the mind. By following the exercise programme in this book – by deepening our connection with the breath and the core – we get in touch with both the physical and spiritual centres of our wellbeing.

"Physical fitness is the first requisite of happiness," wrote Joseph Pilates and it is true that it is very easy to become desperately unhappy if our body cannot function to the best of our ability and fulfil the tasks we hope it will fulfil. While this sounds to a modern ear a little tricky (what about people who cannot, for instance, become athletes?), Pilates actually meant something more sophisticated. Physical fitness, Pilates wrote, is "a uniformly developed body with a sound mind fully capable of naturally, easily, and satisfactorily performing our many and varied daily tasks with spontaneous zest and pleasure." It is, once again, a question of balance. Is our body the best it could be? Do we enjoy it to the max? Is our body able to do the things we need it to do, given proper accommodations and support?

This question of support is actually central to the question of the centre (if you see what I mean). Core strength is key to correct human function: every other movement affects and is affected by the strength of the core. Our arms, our legs and just about everything else is affected by how strong our core is: the core muscles support the spine, the ribs, and those have knock-on effects to everything else. If we work on having a strong core – which we do in every single one of these exercises – we are secretly working on everything else as well. Find your centre; work on your centre; everything else will follow.

Let's lean in to a couple of exercises designed to really work those central muscles.

EXERCISE

All Fours

We come now onto all fours. This exercise really demands that we bring in our core, because we need to unite all four limbs (and also keep the head, neck and spine fully engaged) – so get ready.

Bring your knees about a hip–width apart, with your ankles in line with your knees. Get your wrists under your shoulders, and your hands splayed for support. Stack the wrists and elbows; stack the hips and knees. Press your shins and the tops of your feet into the mat.

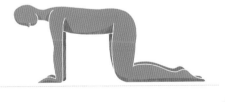

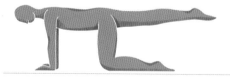

Engage your core, tucking your pelvic muscles in and tightening your abdominal muscles to really support your spine.

Inhale. Exhale, and on the exhale start by pushing the right leg straight out behind you. Point the toes.

Hold. Inhale. Exhale to bring it back down.

Repeat on the left side.

Hold. Inhale. Exhale to bring it back down.

How does that feel?

Let's try the arms now, keeping the ankles and knees stacked and steady.

Inhale. Exhale, and on the exhale push the right arm straight out before you. Point the fingers.

Hold. Inhale. Exhale to bring it back down.

Repeat on the left side.

Hold. Inhale. Exhale to bring it back down.

How does that feel?

Now let's try combining the two: left leg and right arm, both at the same time. Inhale, and exhale to stretch both out. Inhale. Hold for five. Exhale to bring back down.

Maybe you're feeling a bit wobbly here, but that's okay – you will improve! You have time, and practice makes perfect.

Repeat on the other side.

You will probably notice that one side is more wobbly than the other, and that's okay too!

Repeat for ten.

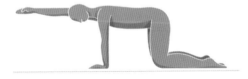

Devote Energy to Yourself

Core strength affects everything in our lives. It's not just a question of a six-pack (!) but of being able to live our lives more efficiently and accurately, and not wasting time and energy on tasks that should be pretty easy. We use our core for almost everything we do, even when we're only sitting still. In fact, a simple way to improve your core strength is to sit up. Right now. Pull your shoulder blades together, tuck your stomach in and sit up nice and tall.

Let's do it: and breathe. In for five, hold for five, out for five. In this way, we can strengthen our core – but we can also form connections. You and I, separated by this book, are also connected by the deep breath we just took together.

You see, core strength helps us but it also helps others. If we turn our attention inward sometimes, we become more productive, happier and stronger members of our community. "Were man to devote as much time and energy to himself as he has devoted to that which man has produced, what astounding and unbelievable progress would be made; a progress eclipsing all he has so far successfully accomplished," wrote Joseph Pilates. In other words, we should pay as much attention to our bodies – the things that make – as we do to the things that we make, and the lives

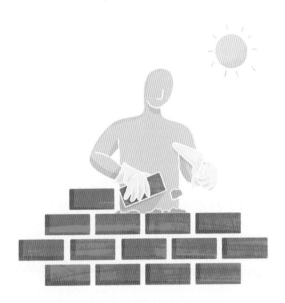

that we build. When we have a strong and happy builder, we can build better. When the builder is unhappy and in pain, we can do nothing.

This is true on every level: physically within the muscles of the body, and within the communities we make, and mentally and spiritually. We have to tend to the core – to the core self – in order that everything else will function correctly.

The Pilates Hundred

The Pilates Hundred is the beginning of almost every Pilates class you will ever take: it's not complicated, and can be done easily at home. It also works nearly every muscle in the body, but especially strengthens the core. You'll also be able to see here quite clearly how the core helps and supports the spine and the limbs.

Don't get worried by the word "hundred": you don't have to do it all at once if you can't manage. Breaks are allowed for beginners! (And, in fact, for anyone else who wants one.)

The name of the exercise comes from the hundred pulses of the arms.

Lie on your back.

Inhale for five.

Bring your legs up to a kind of tabletop position, and exhale for five.

Bring your shoulder blades together, under the heartspace (the upper part of the chest where the heart is located), and scoop your tailbone up off the floor. Notice the hollow created there. Concentrate on that feeling.

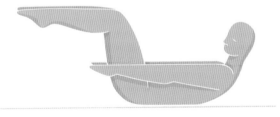

Inhale for five.

Extend your arms and legs, or keep them in tabletop position for an easier variation.

Your arms should be hovering just a couple of inches off the floor. Feel the strain and the pull.

Reeeeeeach with your fingertips.

Now, we're going to speed up the breathing. Instead of in for five and out for five, we will do five short breaths in followed by five short breaths out.

Pulse your arms up and down in time with the breath. Focus on each tiny movement of the arms. Concentrate!

Up down, up down, up down, up down, up down. Five sets of two, an up pulse and a down pulse. Repeat ten times. There you go! That's the Hundred! That's the core!

We call it the core, or the centre, because it's at the heart of everything. The heart of Pilates is in our increased consciousness of that core: spiritually, mentally, physically. We can – and must – bring that awareness into our everyday lives. The modern world seeks to diminish our core strength every day, through the ways we work, travel and live. (Even modern chairs, which are meant to support our bodies, aren't especially helpful!)

So we have to fight for it. We have to remember to pay attention to the core: to bring that concentrated, precise focus to the centre at all hours of the day.

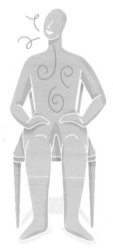

So right now, sit up tall; straighten your back; kiss those shoulder blades together. Tuck that core in. Breathe deep. Breathe tall. Feel the energy flow in with the air, and down deep into your lungs, and out again into the universe.

If you take one thing with you from this book, let it be this moment – and repeat it whenever you can.

Chapter 6:
Flow

" Change happens
through movement,
and movement heals "

– Joseph Pilates

There is something very moving about the simple concept that change is movement, and that movement can heal. The idea that change, which is so frightening to so many of us, might be in fact what heals us, is worth a moment's pause.

There is a famous quotation, from the writer Anaïs Nin, about how painful it can be to remain as a bud when you wish to bloom; and how, however afraid you are of what it will be to blossom, there will come a time when you no longer have a choice. It will be more painful to stay as you are than to simply take the plunge. Change is movement, and movement heals.

Through a sequence of movements, then, we can find a sequence of changes – and this is what we call the flow.

The flow of energy is a huge concept in all our thinking about wellness – from the very ancient to the very modern. Pilates may only have come into being a century ago, but conversations about the flow of energy have been happening for as long as humans have been wondering how to feel better. In ancient Chinese philosophy it's called qi, or life force, and it's known as chi in Buddhism, and these words literally translate to "breath". Yes, we're right back where we started: flow is breath and breath is flow. Breath is energy, and the flow of that breath is the most important thing of all.

Before we explore the importance of flow to Pilates, let's try an ancient Sanskrit technique known as *Nadi Shodhana*. We briefly in the first chapter spoke of *pranayama*, the yogic breathing methods, and this is one of them. It literally means "purification flow" (*nadi*, which means "flow" and *shodhana*, which means "purification") and in English is known as "channel-clearing breath".

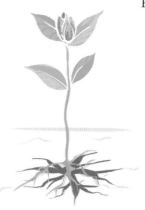

Breath is life; and life is flow. Life is energy, and energy must flow. Blocked energy will cause problems, somewhere down the line.

All wellness comes down to this – and so does science. These are the basic principles of being human.

EXERCISE

Channel-clearing Breath

Sit comfortably. Straight back, neutral spine, core muscles – of course – tucked in. Visualize a clean line from the nape of your neck down to your tailbone. Shoulder blades kiss, as usual.

Put your index finger and your middle finger on your forehead, just above your nose. Cover your right nostril with your thumb. Close your mouth.

For a count of eight, breathe in through your open nostril.

For a count of eight, breathe out through the same open nostril.

Release your right nostril; cover your left nostril with your ring finger.

For a count of eight, breathe in through your open nostril.

For a count of eight, breathe out through the same open nostril.

Repeat for 12 rounds.

Remember, energy is, scientifically speaking, the base matter of the universe. The study of the movement of energy is more usually called the study of physics. We know, for instance, that energy can neither be created nor destroyed. Energy simply transfers from one thing to another, from one being to another, moving through everything in the universe. Take, for instance, something as easy and everyday as making a cup of tea.

When we boil a kettle, the electric energy transfers into the cold water transforming it into hot water and when we tilt the kettle to pour the water the energy from our bodies becomes the energy in the pouring water and the hot water falls onto the teabag, releasing the energy that came from the sun beating down on the leaves of the faraway plant, releasing the flavour, and we drink the tea and our hands are warmed by the heat from the electricity that was generated from the wind or the sun or the long-ago creatures of the earth; and our mind is stimulated by the chemicals created in the leaves of the plant by the sun and the earth. It's all connected; it's all linked; and it flows into us and lets us sit down to write or stretch out on the Pilates mat or pick up a child or tend to a friend or whatever else needs to happen. And then the flow goes on. The energy of the universe is in constant, unbelievable, incredible flux. It moves always and forever and there is no stopping it. Isn't that terrifying? Isn't that amazing to think about?

We can't stop the energy moving through the universe.

We can only try to embrace it.

And it is this embracing it – and trying to better understand how we can flow with the energy rather than against it – that is what makes Pilates so remarkable.

References

[1]   Hofmann, Stefan G. et al. "The effect of mindfulness-based therapy on anxiety and depression: A meta-analytic review". *Journal of Consulting and Clinical Psychology*, Vol. 78, No. 2 (2010), 169–183.

[2]   Walsh, R. and S.L. Shapiro, "The meeting of meditative disciplines and western psychology: A mutually enriching dialogue". *American Psychologist*, 61(3) (2006), 227–239.

[3]   WBessel van der Kolk M D, *The Body Keeps the Score*, Viking Books, 2014.